Me as a Lady, My Well-being, My Sexual coexistence with Cloves

By

Lydia O. Caleb

Copyright ©2023

Chapter by chapter guide

Here are some clove water helps that each well being cognizant individual ought to know about

Further develops processing

Decreases weight

Controls sugar level

Antibacterial properties

Assists with irritation

Advances bone wellbeing

Cloves helps with origination

Helps during Period

Cloves facilitates feminine agony

The most effective method to involve cloves as a sex sugar

Step by step instructions to utilize cloves to treat vagina tingling

- Vaginal Infection

Clove Oil For Infection

- The most effective method to utilize cloves to treat diseases
- Cloves for hack
- Clove oil for the treatment of Scabies
- Cloves for looseness of the bowels
- Cloves for Skin Acne
- Clove oil for hair

Instructions to make Clove oil at home

End

About the book

Me as a lady, my wellbeing, my sexual coexistence with
cloves.
This book is about how ladies can have the option to
deal with their wellbeing and their sexual coexistence
and make their adoration lives more agreeable by
causing their accomplices to request more.
I was nearly losing everything in my sexual life, until I
explored Cloves, then I found a great deal about cloves
and what I can profit from this plant.
Presently concerning my sexual life, it changed
emphatically after I applied this technique that you will
likewise get to be aware in the wake of perusing this
book.
I have given this suggestion to such countless ladies
and they are vouching for it.
It is not difficult to get and I'm sure that we have it in our
kitchens.
Check it out and I want to believe that you give your
audit.
Lydia O. Caleb

Presentation

Clove is a significant flavor and is otherwise called " Nature's Clean".
It is a successful home solution for toothache. You can put an entire clove close to the longing tooth to get help from the aggravation. Clove can assist with giving help from hack and sore throat because of its antimicrobial, cell reinforcement and mitigating properties. It can likewise assist in the administration of diabetes as it can bring down the glucose levels.
Clove oil can likewise assist with forestalling mosquito chomps because of its superb mosquito repellent property.
Cloves can assist with improving sex. It can likewise help with origination and parcels more.

What is cloves

Clove is a flavor that is plentiful in cell reinforcements, nutrients, and minerals. Cloves have been utilized in conventional Chinese medication and Ayurvedic medication to reinforce the resistant framework, lessen irritation, and help in assimilation.

Cloves are obtained from an evergreen tree (Syzygium aromaticum) local to Indonesia. Albeit presently, it is filled in different regions of the planet, like South America
Despite the fact that it was initially a zest utilized for cooking, cloves are turning out to be more well known as elective medication. Become familiar with this intriguing spice and how you can integrate it into your day to day existence.

What Are Ground Cloves?

Ground cloves are a sort of ground flavor that is produced using the dried, ground petals of the clove blossom. They have serious areas of strength for flavor and are utilized in both sweet and exquisite dishes. They are accessible in powdered structure and can be found in all things considered supermarkets.

Entire Versus Ground Cloves

Entire cloves are unground, and ground cloves are the powder that is left after the cloves are ground.

Ground zest can be utilized as a substitute for the entire flavor in many recipes. To supplant 1 teaspoon of entire cloves, use ¾ teaspoon of the powdered flavor as a guideline

The most effective method to Ground

Might you want to make your own hand crafted ground cloves? How it's done:

Begin with the entire clove.

Grind them in a mortar and pestle.
In the event that the cloves are still somewhat
enormous, you can utilize an espresso processor to
make them into a better powder.
Store in a hermetically sealed compartment.

To utilize ground flavors, add them to recipes that call for
different flavors like cinnamon, allspice, and nutmeg.
You can likewise involve them in sweet or exquisite
dishes, or as a topping. Trial and find the ideal
equilibrium for your taste buds!

Benefits

A portion of the primary medical advantages of cloves
are as per the following:

They have calming, pain relieving (torment easing), and
antimicrobial properties.
Clove oil is a characteristic moth repellent.
They are utilized as a food additive.
Clove oil is utilized in fragrant healing to treat respiratory
issues, toothache, and sickness
counting heartburn, and sore throats.
Cloves have for some time been utilized for restorative
purposes, one of which is the sexual benefits of cloves.
That is right, cloves have for quite some time been

utilized as a characteristic solution for improving sexual wellbeing, and this article will examine the advantages of cloves concerning sexual wellbeing.

Supplements in Cloves

Cloves are high in nutrients and minerals, including the accompanying:

Vitamin E
Calcium
Magnesium
Potassium
Iron
Vitamin K
Potassium
Zinc
Folate
Choline and so on.

Likewise, it contains different valuable parts notwithstanding nutrients and minerals, essentially phenolic compounds including;

eugenol,
hydroxyphenyl propane,
hydroxycinnamic corrosive and so forth

flavonoids like quercetin and kaempferol
hydroxybenzoic corrosive,
Phenolic acids principally caffeic ferulic, ellagic, and
salicylic acids.

We should take a gander at the sexual advantages of
cloves since it has become so undeniably obvious what
they are.

Advantages of Cloves Physically for ladies

1. Treatment of general sex medical issues

Cloves have generally been used to treat male sexual
troubles in Ayurvedic and Unani medication due to their
sexual advantages, and furthermore the utilization of
cloves for sex upgrade, explicitly the nerve excitement
and it has additionally been accounted for the sexual
way of behaving supporting impacts of cloves.

Cloves are the most ideal way to treat you in the event that you are managing what is happening as has been seen.

Tip: Applying a cream containing clove oil could be the response.

2. Advance sex chemical creation

As per concentrates on because of cloves on sex chemical profiles, subcutaneous treatment of clove extricate in low measurements works on sexual execution by helping testosterone and prolactin levels.

Cloves are high in manganese, which fills in as a basic controller or trigger of sex chemical creation.

3. Increments anxious excitement

This strong synapse can decrease pulse and initiate the parasympathetic sensory system. This sort of framework is liable for starting an "instinctive" reaction inside the person".

4. Avoidance of sexually transmitted diseases brought about by helpless creatures

Microscopic organisms, infections, and microbes are among the most well-known reasons for physically sent contaminations (STIs), otherwise called Physically Communicated Illnesses (sexually transmitted diseases) (sexually transmitted diseases).

As per a review, "Cloves have antibacterial, antiviral, antifungal, and calming impacts, which might help with the counteraction and treatment of sexually transmitted diseases."

5. Lessens chances of barrenness

Cloves upgrade ovulation in ladies thus lessen barrenness, cloves might further develop sperm quality and subsequently diminish fruitlessness.

"Cloves are a notable richness promoter for all kinds of people and are known to treat male and female fruitlessness. Individuals polish off clove water subsequent to absorbing water to treat fruitlessness and further develop pregnancy."

6. Liver-related sexual brokenness

Patients with liver infection are more inclined to have sexual issues. The compound eugenol, tracked down in cloves, should help with liver issues and sexual brokenness in little doses.

7. Cloves for mouth ulcer

Clove assists with diminishing agony and irritation in the mouth because of its recuperating impact. This is credited to its Katu (sharp), Tikta (unpleasant) and Sita (cold) properties.

Tip:
1. Take 2-5 drops of Clove oil and blend in with 1 teaspoon of Coconut oil.
2. Douse a cotton ball in it.
3. Delicately swipe the ball around the impacted region.
4. Repeat it one time per day.

8. Clove for Butt-centric crevice

Cloves may be valuable in the event of persistent butt-centric gaps. Applying skin cream containing Clove oil fundamentally decreases the resting butt-centric strain in patients experiencing ongoing butt-centric gap. Clove assists with decreasing the gamble of butt-centric gap in light of its Ropan (mending) property.

Suggested Measurements

As indicated by the World Wellbeing Association, the day to day suggested portion of cloves is 2.5 mg/kg body weight.

Clove oil: Around a couple of drops of clove oil ought to do the trick.

Clove powder: Utilize a portion of a teaspoon of clove powder more than once per day, contingent upon your requirements.

Instructions to involve cloves for pimples

1. Clove Powder

a. Take 1/4-1/2 teaspoon of Clove powder.
b. Blend it in with honey and apply on the skin.
c. Allow it to sit for 5-10 minutes.
d. Wash with tepid water.
e. Repeat once per week to control pimples.

2. Clove Oil

A. For pimples
a. Blend 2-5 drops of Clove oil with 1 teaspoon of water.
b. Apply on the impacted regions with the assistance of a q-tip prior to hitting the sack around evening time.
c. Wash with tepid water in the first part of the day to oversee agonizing pimples.

For toothache

Eugenol present in Clove has an antinociceptive impact which helps in restraining the difficult tactile nerves and accordingly helps in overseeing toothache.

Clove gives alleviation in the event of toothache and furthermore diminishes the gamble of different oral contaminations due to its Katu (Sharp) and Tikta (severe) properties.

Tip:
1. Place an entire Clove in your mouth or close to the difficult tooth.
a. Nibble gradually to deliver the oil and don't swallow.
b. Repeat this however many times on a regular basis.

2. Put 2-4 drops of Clove oil onto a cotton ball.
a. Presently put this cotton ball on the impacted region and save it for 30-40 minutes.
b. Repeat 1-2 times each day to get help from toothache.

Utilizations of Clove in food to Accomplish Sexual Advantages

Cloves can be utilized in different courses in your eating regimen, including

Clove Tea: To make a pleasant cup of calming clove tea, add 12 teaspoons of clove powder to bubbling water and stew for 5 to 10 minutes.

Clove seasoned Rice
a. Take 2 cups of rice.
b. Absorb them 3 cups of water for 30 minutes.
c. Presently add 5-6 Cloves and bubble in 3 cups of water for 10 minutes.

d. Presently add the absorbed rice to the Clove water and cook well.

Pumpkin pie: For a rich zesty flavor, add ground cloves to your pumpkin pie.

Lattes: To make fiery lattes, you can add a little grounded clove to it.

Cloves and Period Pains

Clove is a calming flavor that incorporates eugenol, which is useful in lessening period distress. Extreme feminine cycle draining is likewise diminished by utilizing this oil.

Clove for Heaving

Clove could help in processing and is valuable in letting the side effects free from gastric touchiness and retching.

Clove assists with controlling retching and sickness as it further develops processing and lessens gastric touchiness by making a relieving impact due its Sita (cold) and Pitta adjusting properties.

Tips:
1. Bite 1-2 Cloves at whatever point you get the sensation of sickness and regurgitating.

2. Or on the other hand you can utilize a couple of Cloves to make some tea.
3. Drink this tea 1-2 times each day to control regurgitating.

What are the advantages of drinking clove water?

Clove water can help your resistant framework and shield you from illnesses and influenza assuming you drink it each day. Clove water is high in nutrients and minerals that could assist with working on your wellbeing and resistance. Manganese, vitamin k, L-ascorbic acid, calcium, and magnesium are plentiful in them.

Step by step instructions to make cloves water

Clove water is one more incredible method for receiving greatest rewards from this solid zest. Simply absorb two cloves a glass of water and keep it short-term. Drink it first thing while starving.
To make cloves that you can store in a container for quite a long time, get a handful of cloves, soak it in water for 72 hours, channel it and store it in a container and use at whatever point you need to.

Here are some clove water helps that each well being cognizant individual ought to know about

Further develops assimilation

The most known advantage of drinking clove water is to help the assimilation interaction. Only one cup of clove water can assist with further developing spit creation that is fundamental for launching the assimilation cycle.

It can likewise increment gastric discharges and decrease side effects related with stomach torment, overabundance gas, and acid reflux.

Lessens weight

One more famous area of clove water benefits is in lessening weight. Solid absorption and rapid digestion are the keys with regards to shedding those difficult kilos.
Clove water assists with further developing assimilation and lift metabolic rate. It works like sorcery in holding your stomach back from snarling between dinners.

Controls sugar level

Anybody watching out for their glucose level will be glad to realize this advantage of drinking clove water.

Research has shown that specific mixtures in clove assist with advancing insulin creation, which, thusly, brings down glucose. Along these lines clove water benefits diabetic patients gigantically.

Antibacterial properties

Clove water benefits reach out to the area of oral cleanliness too. Clove has been explored as an antibacterial specialist for starter research.

In one review, a mouth flush containing clove was found to assist with battling plaque and microorganisms in the mouth.

Whenever joined with legitimate oral cleanliness, the antibacterial properties of clove water can assist with fortifying your oral wellbeing.

Assists with irritation

Cloves are known for their mitigating impacts. Wealthy in cell reinforcements, they can assist you with decreasing oxidative pressure and aggravation. Clove water benefits patients with joint pain more and is particularly prescribed to them.

Advances bone wellbeing

Polishing off clove water consistently can likewise advance bone wellbeing. As we age, we are more in danger of creating undesirable bone diseases like osteoporosis. Clove water benefits us by decreasing such gambling.

The compound in clove can assist with safeguarding bone mass, increment bone thickness, and strength. Likewise an astounding wellspring of manganese is essential for generally speaking bone wellbeing.

Cloves helps with origination

Drinking clove water is accepted to support ovulation and builds a lady's possibilities of origination. Numerous ladies are attempting to consider taking clove water to help ovulation. Cloves are accepted to expand the emission of LH. LH is the chemical that animates the ovaries to deliver eggs during ovulation and feminine cycle.

Helps during Feminine cycle

Clove oil gives quick help from feminine spasms and abbreviates the length of period. Clove is a mitigating flavor as it contains eugenol, which is very advantageous to facilitate the side effects of the period. This oil likewise restricts unreasonable feminine dying.

Cloves facilitates feminine torment

It has been found that knead treatment might assist with lessening the seriousness of period cramps. However, kneading with natural balms saw a more noteworthy decrease of torment. Another preliminary utilized stomach rub with a blend of rejuvenating oils including cinnamon, clove, rose, and lavender in almond oil.

The most effective method to involve cloves as a sex sweetener

For the people who generally gripe that they loath sex or don't have encourage for sex, low moxie, a few ladies will try and say that, in view of how poor their sex making is, that their mates will typically let them know regardless of whether they stand stripped before them it makes next to no difference to them, no desire, no nervousness.

Additionally for the individuals who abhor sex, you are simply doing it just to satisfy your accomplice, no fulfillment toward the finish, all things considered, no pleasantness, no climax.

Here is your answer, set up this beverage and take it generally, in something like fourteen days you will affirm and you will be singing another melody.

It is additionally excellent for dryness of the vagina and sweet aroma from the vagina.

Fixings:

Watermelon, Cloves powder, Fluid milk, Honey and Coconut.

Watermelon:

Watermelon is wealthy in L-citrulline, an amino corrosive that further develops blood stream like Viagra, L-citrulline increments bloodstream to the sexual organs yet with next to no bad aftereffects. Watermelon assumes a basic part in loosening up veins, so bloodstream improves and learns to expect the unexpected. It allows a superior opportunity of useful erection and incredible drive for sex.(Your companion isn't likewise forgotten about).

Get a watermelon, cut off the rear of the watermelon, presently cleave the organic product in more modest sizes with the seeds inside it. Promptly you're finished, blend to get the juice.

Clove:

It assists with supporting one's energy levels. It likewise has one of the most mind-blowing fragrant healing aromas that works on your sexual way of behaving and increases sex drive and invigorates sexual execution.

You can get the powdered one from the store to keep away from the pressure of crushing it.

Coconut:

Coconut is known as a significant cancer prevention agent that safeguards the cells and animates and reinforces conceptive capabilities in people. In a clinical report, ladies in their mid-sixties detailed an expansion in their drive subsequent to drinking coconut water.

Get a coconut, eliminate the hard shell, cut into pieces and get it washed appropriately. Mix the coconut and eliminate the shaft. Guarantee each different fixings are amounted to the coconut
water and mix together.
Put this combination inside a holder and refrigerate for certain minutes before you drink it.

This drink gives the most extreme fulfillment for your sexual coexistence.

The subsequent strategy is the bubbling technique:

Furthermore, there are ideal elements for it.
Sugarcane
Cloves
Ginger
Honey.

Boil Sugarcane, Cloves, Ginger and Honey for like 30 minutes and let it cool. You can accept it as water, it builds Vagina Dampness and empowers you to fulfill your accomplice.

The third strategy:

Here all you want is clove water, squeezed orange and honey.
Combine this as one and drink this combination 30 minutes prior to meeting with your accomplice.

Note: These blends increment Vagina Liquid, Helps dependable sex, makes sex agreeable and furthermore supports your sexual resistant framework and charisma.

Step by step instructions to utilize cloves to treat vagina tingling

Vagina Infection

Vagina infection is many times an intense battle for ladies, particularly the individuals who don't have the foggiest idea about this straightforward approach to treating and warding it off.

It is a typical condition that most ladies experience.

As a matter of fact, concentrate on showing that 75% of ladies are probably going to have no less than one yeast infection during their lifetime.

Numerous ladies experience repetitive vaginal disease, particularly when they open themselves to the reason once more.

The most widely recognized sorts of vagina disease are bacterial and yeast infections.

Vaginal yeast infections are the second most normal reason for strange vaginal release in the US (the first is bacterial vaginosis).

Because of the commonness of vaginal disease, scientists looked for a method for assisting ladies with defeating this terrible experience.

One of the plants that accompany trust for each lady who has vaginal disease is clove.
Also, this is the way you can utilize it, take cloves of water and wash your vaginal morning and night.
Also, in no less than fourteen days you will be fine in the future and continuously feeling revived.

Clove Oil For Infections

Additionally, clove oil is accessible for treatment of infections.

Strangely, clove oil is accessible in various sizes.

Get the oil and drop a couple of it on your gasp liner before you wear your jeans.

The most effective method to utilize cloves to treat diseases

To treat infections, you should consolidate cloves with different plants to obtain a decent outcome.
These are the things you will have to get to obtain the best result.
You will be merging them together and they are
-Cloves
-Ginger
-Garlic
-Turmeric.

Presently here is the technique:

Get a container, fill it with water, dice the tumeric, ginger and garlic, put it in the container loaded up with water alongside the cloves, cover with the top and drench for 72 hours. Begin savoring it in the morning and night, and the portion is around 50% of a glass cup, at the crack of dawn and last thing before sleep time.

Cloves for hack

Eugenol and flavonoids present in Clove have cancer prevention agent, calming, antimicrobial movement and hinder the development of microscopic organisms, infection and yeast. It additionally goes about as an expectorant because of the Kapha and Pitta adjusting properties and it helps in ousting bodily fluid from the respiratory section. This decreases aggravation and assists in making do with hacking.

Tip:
1. Take 1/4 gm of Clove powder.
2. Bubble it in 125ml water till the volume diminishes to 1/fourth.
3. Strain the arrangement and consume when it is still warm.

Tip:
Bite 1-2 Cloves with salt around evening time prior to hitting the hay.

Clove oil for the treatment of Scabies

Clove oil has powerful antimicrobial, cell reinforcement and sedative properties that can be utilized in different ways to oversee Scabies. It is critical to utilize it cautiously and can inflict any kind of damage in the event that it is not weakened with a transporter oil or cream. A few manners by which it tends to be utilized are:

1. Add a drop of Clove oil to a small bunch of lotion/cream and apply to the impacted region.

2. Add 5-6 drops of Clove oil to hot shower water and absorb this water for around 20 minutes.

3. Consolidate 10 drops of Clove oil with 1 teaspoon of honey and 1 teaspoon of coconut oil. Rub it onto the impacted region two times every day.

Cloves for loose bowels

Clove oil could help in processing as it has a germicidal impact against different microscopic organisms like E.coli. It assists in the disposal of parasites and controls with losing movements and heartburn. It is likewise helpful in freeing the side effects from the runs, gastric touchiness and heaving.

Clove assists with controlling the runs as it assists with quieting the gastrointestinal system because of its Deepan (canapé) and Pachan (stomach related) properties which additionally assists with lessening Ama and making the stool thick.

Tips:
1. Take 4 cups of water.
2. Add 1/2 teaspoon Clove.

3. Bubble for 10-15 minutes.
4. Allow it to cool to room temperature and afterward add 1 teaspoon of honey.
5. Drink it two times every day.

Tip:
Blend 2-3 drops of Clove oil in water and drink after a quick bite.

Cloves for Skin Acne

Clove has antibacterial properties and successfully kills cells and biofilms of microorganisms S.aureus which causes skin inflammation.
Clove oil assists with controlling skin inflammation because of its antimicrobial impact. This is because of its Katu (Sharp) and Tikta (unpleasant) properties. Clove additionally further develops twisted mending because of its Ropan (recuperating) property.

Tip:
1. Take 2-3 drops of Clove oil and blend in with 1 teaspoon honey.
2. Apply this on the face and delicately rub with your fingertips.

Clove oil for hair

Indeed, Clove oil is really great for hair when kneaded well on the scalp. It further develops hair development by expanding blood dissemination to the roots. It additionally has insecticidal movement because of its synthetic constituents like eugenol, isoeugenol and methyl eugenol. These substance constituents help in eliminating lice.
Clove assists with forestalling balding because of dandruff and dryness. This is because of its Snigdha (slick) and Katu (impactful) nature. Clove likewise elevates hair development because of its Ropan (recuperating) property.

Instructions to make Clove oil at home

To make Clove oil at home:

1. Put 1 teaspoon of entire Cloves in a container over medium intensity and saute for a couple of moments.
2. Gather the Cloves in a mortar and pestle.

3. Add 1 teaspoon of olive into it and pulverize the Cloves.
4. You can dunk a cotton bud into the oil and use it straightforwardly for toothache or sore gums.
5. You can likewise pour the oil in a dull glass container and store at room temperature.

End

Cloves are advantageous to all kinds of people's sexual wellbeing. It has cancer prevention agent, against microbial, hostile to parasitic, against viral, hostile to nociceptive, immunomodulatory, and hostile to cancer-causing properties, and it increments drive, brain feeling, sperm count, sperm motility, and general sexual wellbeing properties.

9 798376 236215